CANCER DIET
COOKBOOK *FOR* Beginners

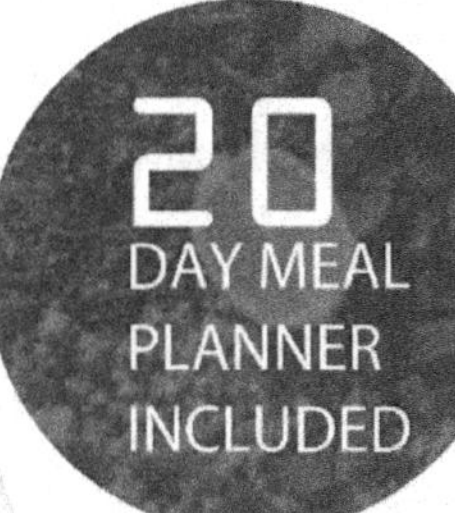

SIMPLE AND DELICIOUS RECIPES FOR CANCER PATIENTS

Cathryn D. Dutton

ABSTRACT

The "Cancer Diet Cookbook for Beginners" is a thorough and approachable manual created for those looking to adopt a regulated or cancer-preventive diet. This painstakingly created cookbook offers a wide variety of dishes that have been carefully selected to provide readers a realistic grasp of how dietary choices can affect their health. Every recipe, from filling breakfast alternatives to fulfilling dinner options, flawlessly combines culinary creativity with nutritional knowledge based on scientific research. The user-friendly design of the cookbook ensures that anyone interested in healthy cuisine may start their journey to wellbeing with confidence. This cookbook is an essential resource for fostering wellness through the enjoyment of delectable, cancer-preventive meals because it places an emphasis on whole ingredients, balanced nutrition, and gourmet combinations. This cookbook invites you to set out on a delectable journey in the direction of a healthier, more energetic future, regardless of your level of cooking experience.

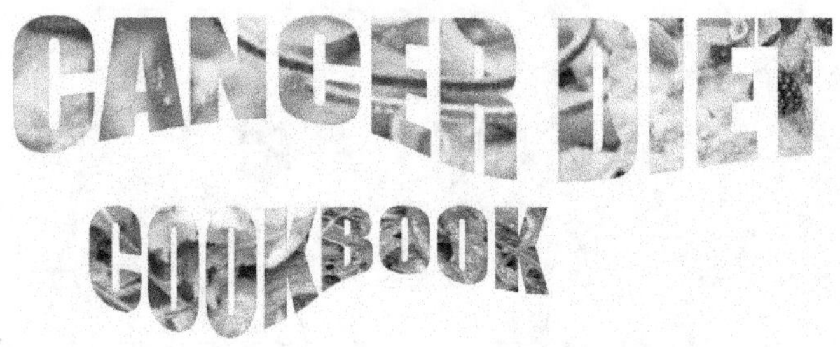

TABLE OF CONTENT

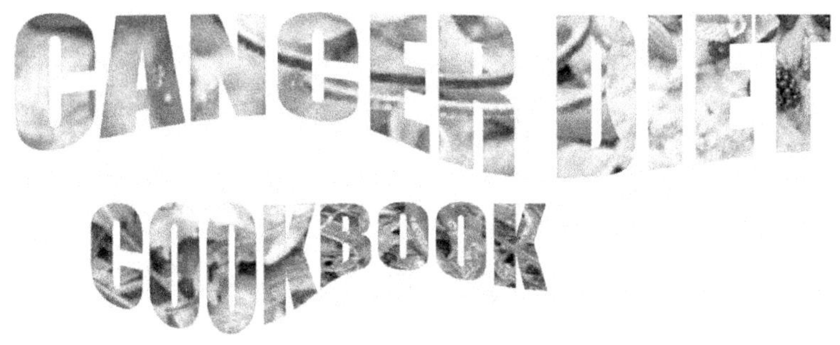
CANCER DIET
COOKBOOK

CANCER DIET
COOKBOOK *FOR* Beginners

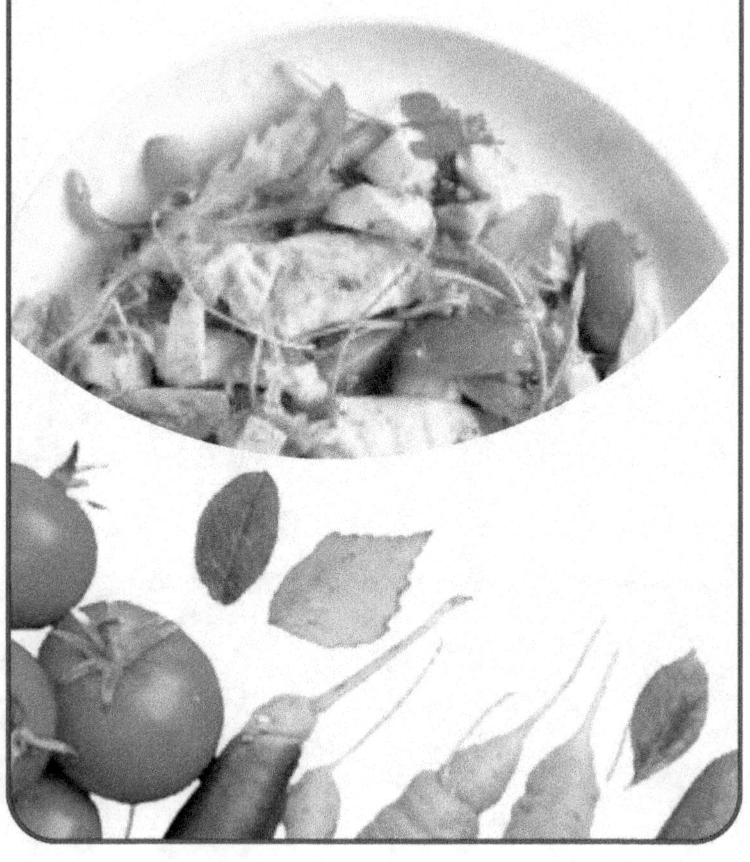

INTRODUCTION

Robert, a resolute person with a strong will, started on a transformational journey as he read through the "Cancer Diet Cookbook for Beginners." Robert was initially intimidated by the idea of changing his eating habits, but his dedication to his health motivated him to move on. He was enthralled by the abundance of gastronomic opportunities that lay ahead of him with each page turn.

Robert enjoyed the process of choosing healthy foods, learning new culinary methods, and creating meals that not only pampered his body but also his taste buds as he made his way through the cookbook.

He gained a fresh appreciation for colorful fruit, lean proteins, and inventive flavor combinations thanks to the cookbook's intelligent advice.

Robert saw improvements in his energy levels, general wellbeing, and even his outlook on life as a result of his efforts over time. His trusted friend, the cookbook, helped him make more informed decisions and live a healthier lifestyle.

Robert's transformation into a skilled cook, fuelled by the information learned through the cookbook, was evidence of his will to actively manage his health and to embrace a more promising, cancer-preventive future.

I am aware of cancer, yes. It is a set of illnesses characterized by the body's aberrant cells growing and spreading out of control. There are several cancers, such as those of the breast, lungs, prostate, and other organs. Depending on the type, symptoms can vary, but typical warning signs include unexplained weight loss, exhaustion, pain, skin abnormalities, and persistent coughing or hoarseness.

Adopting a healthy lifestyle, such as abstaining from tobacco and excessive alcohol use, eating a balanced diet, exercising regularly, protecting your skin from too much sun exposure, and getting regular screenings based on your age and risk factors, are frequently included in cancer prevention strategies. A healthcare expert should be consulted for specific recommendations and advice.

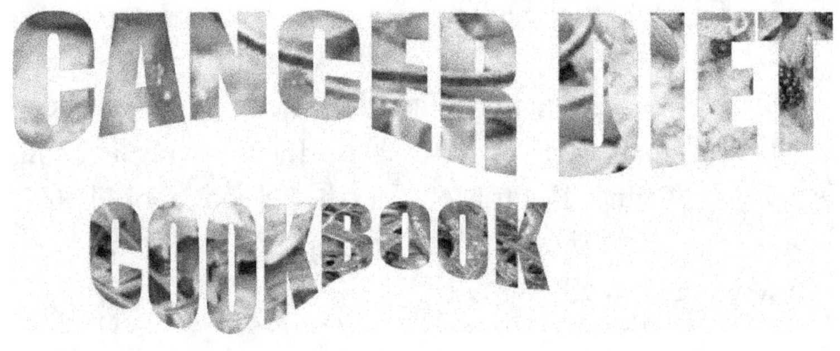

here are 10 breakfast recipes that can be included in a cancer-preventive or controlled diet cookbook for beginners:

1.Oatmeal with Berries

Ingredients

- rolled oats, 1 cup
- 2 cups of water or milk
- A dash of salt
- Strawberry, blueberry, and raspberry-filled 1 cup of mixed berries
- 2 teaspoons of maple syrup or honey
- (Optional) 1/4 cup chopped nuts

Preparation

1. Oats and a dash of salt should be added after simmering milk or water in a saucepan.

2. Over medium heat, cook the oats, stirring regularly, until they are fully cooked and creamy.

3. Serving the oatmeal in dishes with chopped nuts, mixed fruit, and honey or maple syrup on the side is customary.

2. Greek Yogurt Parfait

Ingredients

- Greek yogurt, one cup
- 14 cup of granola
- 1/2 cup of mixed fresh fruits (kiwi, berries, and bananas) Honey, two tablespoons a smidge of vanilla extract

Preparation

1. Layer Greek yogurt, granola, and a variety of fresh fruits in a glass or bowl.

2. Over the layers, drizzle honey and vanilla extract.

3. Once or twice more, repeat the layers, then finish with a granola garnish on top.

3. Avocado Toast

Ingredients

- Whole-grain bread, two pieces 1 mature avocado pepper and salt as desired Flakes of red pepper (optional) cherry tomatoes, sliced (optional) juice of fresh lemons

Preparation

1. The bread pieces should be toasted till golden brown.

2. In a bowl, mash the ripe avocado and add salt, pepper, and a squeeze of fresh lemon juice for flavor.

3. Over the toasted bread, evenly distribute the avocado mixture.

4. If preferred, add sliced cherry tomatoes and red pepper flakes as a garnish.

4. Spinach and Mushroom Scramble

Ingredients

- 3 eggs
- fresh spinach leaves, 1 cup Sliced mushrooms in a cup onion, diced, 14 cup pepper and salt as desired grated cheese, if desired 1 tablespoon of oil or butter

Preparation

1. Butter or oil should be heated in a skillet over medium heat.

2. Sauté the mushrooms until they are soft after adding the diced onion and mushrooms.

3. Cook the added spinach until it wilts.

4. Salt and pepper the eggs in a bowl after beating them, then pour them into the skillet.

5. Gently stir the eggs and vegetables together until they are cooked to your satisfaction.

6. Before serving, grate some cheese if you like.

5. Quinoa Breakfast Bowl

Ingredients

- cooked quinoa, 1 cup
- Fruits (apple, banana, and berries) in a 1/2 cup, diced
- Almonds or chia seeds, in 2 teaspoons, chopped
- 1 tablespoon yogurt or honey Milk splash (optional)

Preparation

1. Place cooked quinoa, diced fruit, and chopped nuts or seeds in a bowl.

2. Yogurt or honey can be drizzled over top.

3. If more creaminess is desired, add a splash of milk.

6. Chia Seed Pudding

Ingredients

- Chia seeds, 1/4 cup
- 1 cup milk, either dairy or vegan
- 1 tablespoon of maple syrup or honey One-half teaspoon of vanilla extract fresh fruit as a garnish

Preparation

1. Chia seeds, milk, honey, or maple syrup, and vanilla essence should be combined in a jar or other container.

2. Once thoroughly combined, the mixture should be chilled for at least a few hours or overnight to thicken.

3. Give it a thorough swirl before serving, and then top with fresh fruit.

7. Smoked Salmon Wrap

Ingredients

- 1 tortilla whole-wheat a few slices of smoked salmon a serving of cream cheese, two sliced red onion, thin Capers
- recent dill

Preparation

1. On a spotless surface, spread out the whole wheat tortilla.

2. Over the tortilla, evenly spread cream cheese.

3. Then arrange the smoked salmon pieces on top of the cream cheese.

4. Over the salmon, scatter capers and red onion that has been finely sliced.

5. Add some fresh dill as garnish.

6. The tortilla should be securely rolled, then sliced in half diagonally and served.

8. Berry Smoothie

Ingredients

- Strawberry, blueberry, and raspberry-filled 1 cup of mixed berries one banana
- 1 cup milk, either dairy or vegan
- Greek yogurt, half a cup
- 1 tablespoon of maple syrup or honey
- Several ice cubes

Preparation

1. Blend the mixed berries, banana, milk, Greek yogurt, honey, or maple syrup, and ice cubes in a blender until smooth.

2. Blend till creamy and smooth.

3. Enjoy the smoothie by pouring it into glasses.

9. Whole Grain Pancakes

Ingredients

- whole wheat flour, 1 cup 1 teaspoon of sugar one tablespoon of baking powder A half-teaspoon of baking soda

- Salt: 1/4 teaspoon; buttermilk: 1 cup
- 1 egg
- melted butter, two tablespoons Fresh berries as a garnish

1. Combine whole wheat flour, sugar, baking soda, baking powder, and salt in a mixing bowl.

2. Whisk the buttermilk, egg, and melted butter in a separate basin.

3. Mix the dry ingredients just until mixed after adding the wet ingredients.

4. Butter or oil should be used to lightly coat a skillet or griddle before heating it up.

5. For each pancake, pour 1/4 cup of the batter into the skillet.

6. Cook until surface bubbles appear, then turn and continue to cook the other side until golden.

7. Put fresh berries on top of the pancakes before serving.

10. Fruit Salad with Nuts

Ingredients

- a variety of fresh fruits (oranges, grapes, kiwis, melon, pineapple) mixed nuts (almonds, walnuts, and cashews) in 1/4 cup mint leaves for garnish, fresh For drizzling, use honey or lime juice

Preparation

1. The fresh fruits should be washed, peeled, and cut into bite-sized pieces.

2. In a bowl, combine the diced fruits.

3. To the bowl, add the mixed nuts.

4. Sprinkle lime juice or honey over the fruit and almonds.

5. Gently blend by tossing.

6. Use fresh mint leaves as a garnish.

7. Immediately serve the fruit salad.

Enjoy your delicious and nutritious breakfast!

Just keep in mind that you can adjust these recipes to suit your tastes and dietary requirements. For individualized dietary advice, always seek the advice of a medical practitioner..

Here are 10 lunch recipes suitable for a cancer-preventive or controlled diet cookbook for beginners:

1. Grilled Chicken Salad

Ingredients

- shaved-bone chicken breasts
- mixed salad greens, such as lettuce, spinach, and arugula
- Cherry tomatoes, split cucumbers, thinly cut bell peppers, sliced red onions, and sliced olive oil
- Citrus juice
- Pepper and salt
- Nuts, seeds, cheese, and your choice of dressing are optional additions.

Preparation

1. Chicken breasts should be marinated in olive oil, lemon juice, salt, and pepper. Cook completely on the grill.

2. Slice the chicken after letting it rest.

3. Salad greens, cherry tomatoes, cucumber, red onion, and bell peppers should all be combined in a big bowl.

4. On top, scatter the cooked chicken slices.

5. Add additional lemon juice and olive oil to taste. Add salt and pepper to taste. Dressing and additional toppings are optional. Serve after gently tossing.

2. Quinoa and Vegetable Stir-Fry

Ingredients

- Quinoa
- Mixed veggies (such as bell peppers, carrots, and broccoli), minced, and chopped onion and garlic
- sour cream soybean oil grated ginger
- Pepper and salt
- Elective: tofu, nuts, and seeds

Preparation

1. Quinoa should be prepared as directed on the packaging. Place aside.

2. Sesame oil should be heated in a big pan or wok. Mix in the chopped ginger, garlic, and onion. until fragrant, sauté.

3. Stir-fry the added vegetables in a mixture until they begin to soften.

4. Add soy sauce and salt & pepper to taste.

5. Stir-fry everything together after adding cooked quinoa to the pan.

6. Add tofu, nuts, or seeds as an optional addition for more texture and protein. Once thoroughly heated, turn off the heat and serve.

3. Mediterranean Wrap

Ingredients

- Whole wheat tortillas or wraps
- Hummus
- Chicken kabobs or falafel
- Sliced Kalamata olives, sliced cucumber, tomato, red onion, pitted and diced feta cheese, and crumbled
- Olive oil, chopped fresh parsley
- Citrus juice
- Pepper and salt

Preparation

1. The wraps should be set out with a layer of hummus on each.

2. Each wrap should have grilled chicken or falafel in the middle.

3. Add olives, feta cheese, cucumber, tomato, red onion, and parsley as garnishes.

4. Lemon juice and olive oil should be drizzled on. Add salt and pepper to taste.

5. The wrap's sides should be folded in and rolled up tightly.

6. Before serving, if necessary, secure with toothpicks and cut in half diagonally.

4. Tomato Basil Soup

Ingredients

- ripe tomatoes, minced, chopped onion, and minced garlic chopped vegetables, new basil leaves, or chicken broth
- Almond oil
- Pepper and salt Heavy cream is optional.

Preparation

1. In a big pot, heat the olive oil. Onion and garlic should be added and sautéed until transparent.

2. Cook the tomatoes, in chunks, until the juices are released.

3. Add the broth, then bring the dish to a boil. Turn down the heat, cover, and simmer for about 20 minutes.

4. Until the soup is creamy, purée it using an immersion blender. Alternately, allow the soup to cool a little before

5. blending it in small batches using a standard blender.

6. Put the soup back in the pot. Add the basil leaves, chopped.

7. Add a little heavy cream, if using, for a creamier texture.

8. To taste, add salt and pepper to the food. If necessary, reheat the soup one more before serving.

5. Lentil Salad

Ingredients

- Green, brown, or French lentils that have been cooked, cooled Cucumber, sliced Red bell pepper, diced Red onion, and finely chopped Cherry tomatoes, cut in half.
- Lemon juice, diced Feta cheese, and fresh parsley
- Almond oil
- Pepper and salt

Preparation

1. Cooked lentils, sliced cucumber, diced red bell pepper, diced red onion, split cherry tomatoes, chopped parsley, and crumbled feta cheese should all be combined in a big bowl.

2. Lemon juice and olive oil should be drizzled on. Add salt and pepper to taste.

3. Gently toss the salad to include all the ingredients and distribute the dressing.

4. If necessary, taste and adjust the seasoning.

5. Before serving, let the lentil salad cool for about 30
    minutes in the fridge.

6. Brown Rice Bowl with Salmon

Ingredients

- Finished brown rice Filet of salmon sour cream soybean
  oil Citrus juice minced garlic various vegetables
  (including carrots, bell peppers, and broccoli) pepper
  and salt as desired
- Optional garnishes: green onions, sesame seeds

Preparation

1. Soy sauce, sesame oil, lemon juice, and minced garlic
    are combined to create a marinade for the salmon fillet.
    Allow it to marinade for 20 to 30 minutes.

2. Set a skillet to medium-high heat to pre-heat. The salmon
    fillet should be cooked through after a few minutes on
    each side.

3. The various vegetables should be stir-fried in the same
    skillet until they are crisp-tender.

4. To assemble, add cooked salmon, stir-fried vegetables, and any additional toppings you choose to a dish of cooked

5. brown rice. If you'd like, add more soy sauce or lemon juice.

7. Chickpea and Vegetable Curry

Ingredients

- chickpeas (cooked or in a can)
- Vegetables in a mixture, such as potatoes, carrots, and peas chopped onion, minced garlic, minced ginger Curry paste or powder coconut cream Plant-based broth
- Tomato sauce Almond oil pepper and salt as desired garnish with fresh cilantro

Preparation

1. Olive oil is heated over medium heat in a big pot. Add the minced ginger, minced garlic, and onion. Once the onions are transparent and fragrant, sauté.

2. Add tomato paste and curry powder or paste. Cooking releases the flavors after a little period of time.

3. Add chickpeas and a mixture of vegetables. To thoroughly distribute the spices, stir well.

4. Vegetable broth and coconut milk should be added. Simmer the vegetables until they are ready.

5. To taste, add salt and pepper to the food.

6. Garnish the curry with fresh cilantro and serve it over rice or naan bread.

8. Tuna Salad Lettuce Wraps

Ingredients

- drained Greek yogurt, mayonnaise, or canned tuna
- The Dijon mustard
- Red onion, coarsely cut, chopped celery, and chopped pickles
- pepper and salt as desired Leaves of lettuce

Preparation

1. Drained tuna, Greek yogurt or mayonnaise, Dijon mustard, diced celery, sliced red onion, and chopped pickles should all be combined in a bowl.

2. Blend thoroughly. Depending on your taste, add salt and pepper to the dish.

3. Place a spoonful of the tuna salad mixture on each lettuce leaf.

4. To make wraps, roll up the lettuce leaves. If required, secure with toothpicks.

5. The tuna salad wraps can be served as a light and energizing lunch.

9. Roasted Veggie Quinoa Bowl

Ingredients

- washed and cooked quinoa
- a variety of veggies (including cherry tomatoes, bell peppers, red onions, and zucchini) Almond oil vinegar of balsam clove powder
- pepper and salt as desired
- Fresh herbs (such basil and parsley), along with optional chopped feta cheese

Preparation

- Preheat the oven to 400°F (200°C).

- Combine the olive oil, balsamic vinegar, garlic powder, salt, and pepper with the assortment of veggies.

- On a baking sheet, spread out the vegetables, and roast them in a preheated oven until they are soft and have developed a mild caramelization.

- Place the cooked quinoa in the bottom of the bowl, then add the roasted veggies, fresh herbs, and, if wanted, the crumbled feta cheese.

10. Vegetable and Bean Soup

Ingredients

- (Cooked or canned) mixed beans a variety of veggies (including bell peppers, carrots, and celery) chopped onion minced garlic Plant-based broth chopped tomatoes in a can
- Italian spices a bay leaf Almond oil pepper and salt as desired garnishing with fresh parsley

Preparation

1. Olive oil is heated over medium heat in a big pot. Add minced garlic and onion, chopped. Sauté onions until they are transparent.

2. Add the additional vegetables and continue to sauté for a few minutes.

3. Add tomato dices from a can of tomato broth. Add bay leaves and Italian seasoning. Simmer for a while.

4. Fill the pot with the mixed beans. The soup should be simmered until the veggies are soft and the flavors are well-balanced.

5. After removing the bay leaves, season the soup to taste
    with salt and pepper. Hot vegetable and bean soup
    should be served with fresh parsley on top.

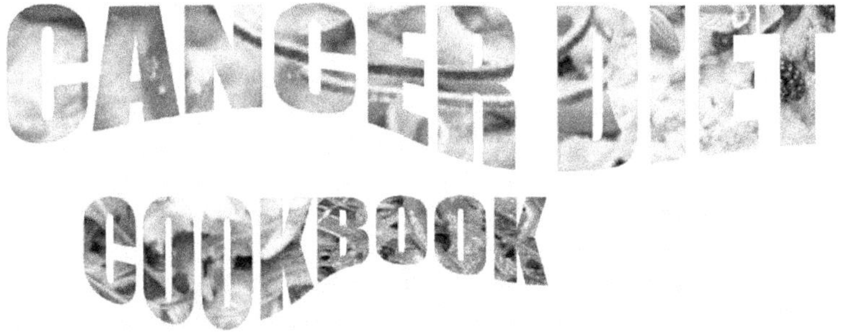

CANCER DIET
COOKBOOK *FOR* Beginners

Certainly! Here are 10 dinner recipes suitable for a cancer-preventive or controlled diet cookbook for beginners:

1. Salmon baked in the oven with steamed vegetables

Ingredients

- Filet of salmon
- various vegetables (including carrots, broccoli, and zucchini)
- EVOO, LEMON JUICE
- Pepper and salt herbs (such as parsley or dill)

Preparation

1. Preheat the oven to 400°F (200°C).

2. On a baking sheet, place the salmon fillet and top with olive oil, lemon juice, salt, pepper, and fresh herbs.

3. The salmon should be baked for 15 to 20 minutes, or until it is thoroughly cooked and flakes with a fork.

4. Steam the various vegetables until they are soft while the salmon is baking.

5. Steamed veggies should be served alongside the baked salmon.

2.Grilled Chicken with Quinoa and Roasted Veggies: Ingredients

- chicken thigh Quinoa
- various vegetables (including red onion, bell peppers, and zucchini)
- EVOO with garlic powder Pepper and salt vinegar of balsam

Preparation

1. For around 30 minutes, marinate the chicken breast in olive oil, garlic powder, salt, and pepper.

2. The grill or grill pan should be preheated to medium-high heat.

3. Grill the chicken for 6 to 8 minutes on each side, or until thoroughly done.

4. Cook the quinoa per the directions on the package while the chicken is roasting.

5. Combine the olive oil, salt, and pepper with the assortment of veggies. They should be baked at 400°F (200°C) until they are soft and have developed a light caramel color.

6. With the roasted vegetables on the side, plate the grilled chicken over cooked quinoa. Add a balsamic vinegar drizzle.

3. Stir-Fried Tofu and Broccoli

Ingredients

- Cubed, firm tofu cauliflower florets sour cream soybean oil
- minced ginger and garlic Flakes of red pepper (optional)
- a mixture of soy sauce, hoisin sauce, and rice vinegar used as a stir-fry sauce

Preparation

1. Sesame oil is added to a skillet or wok that is heated at medium-high heat.

2. Tofu cubes are added and stir-fried until just beginning to color. Take out of the pan and place aside.

3. Sauté the minced ginger, garlic, and red pepper flakes (if using) for a minute in a little more sesame oil in the same pan.

4. Broccoli florets should be added and stir-fried until tender-crisp.

5. Add the stir-fry sauce and mix everything to coat before adding the tofu back to the pan.

6. Over rice or noodles, plate the stir-fried tofu and broccoli.

4. Whole-Wheat Pasta with Tomato and Basil Sauce

Ingredients

- Whole grain pasta chopped tomatoes
- chopped garlic, fresh basil leaves, and olive oil
- Pepper and salt
- Parmesan cheese, grated (optional)

Preparation

1. Follow the directions on the package to prepare the whole-wheat pasta. Drain, then set apart.

2. Olive oil is heated in a skillet at a medium temperature. When aromatic, add the minced garlic and sauté for one minute.

3. Cook the diced tomatoes after adding them until their juices begin to come out.

4. Basil leaves, salt, and pepper are stirred in. For a few minutes, simmer.

5. Combine the tomato and basil sauce with the cooked pasta.

6. If preferred, top with grated Parmesan cheese while serving.

5. Baked Sweet Potato with Black Beans and Salsa

Ingredients

- The sweet potato drained and washed black beans (Homemade or store-bought) salsa (Optional) Greek yogurt or sour cream chopped cilantro, if desired.

Preparation

1. Set the oven's temperature to 400°F (200°C).

2. The sweet potatoes should be washed, forked, and put on a baking pan.

3. The sweet potatoes should be baked for 45 to 60 minutes, or until they are soft.

4. In a microwave or a saucepan, warm the black beans.

5. Cut open the baked sweet potatoes, then use a fork to fluff the interiors.

6. Each sweet potato should have black beans, salsa, and, if preferred, a dollop of sour cream or Greek yogurt on top.

7. Add some chopped cilantro.

Enjoy your delicious meals!

6. Veggie and Lentil Stew

Ingredients

- cup of drained and rinsed green or brown lentils
- peeled and sliced carrots
- 2 chopped celery stalks
- 1 diced onion, 3 minced garlic cloves
- 1 tomato diced can
- 4 cups of veggie broth
- 2 cups of assorted, finely cut veggies, such as bell peppers, zucchini, and spinach
- 1/9 cup cumin 1 paprika teaspoon pepper and salt as desired
- For garnish, use fresh parsley or cilantro.

Preparation

1. Saute celery, carrots, and onions in a big pot until the onions are transparent.

2. Add the paprika, cumin, and garlic. Cook for an additional minute.

3. Vegetable broth, diced tomatoes, and lentils should be added. After bringing to a boil, turn down the heat, cover, and simmer for about 20 minutes.

4. When the lentils and veggies are cooked, add the mixed vegetables and simmer for an additional 10-15 minutes.

5. Add salt and pepper to taste.
6. Serve the stew hot with fresh cilantro or parsley on top.

7. Grilled Veggie and Hummus Wrap

Ingredients

- tacos made with whole wheat
- a variety of grilled veggies, including bell peppers, zucchini, and eggplant
- Hummus
- fresh lettuce or spinach Very thinly sliced red onion
- Feta cheese, if desired Almond oil pepper and salt as desired

1. Preparation
2. Salt and pepper the grilled vegetables, then grill them until they are soft and just beginning to sear. Brush with olive oil.

3. Place a whole wheat tortilla on the table and cover it with a thick layer of hummus.

4. Over the hummus, scatter some fresh spinach or lettuce.

5. On top of the greens, arrange the grilled vegetables.

6. If desired, incorporate some red onion slices and feta cheese crumbles.

7. To make a wrap, roll up the tortilla and tuck the sides in.

8.Cauliflower Rice Stir-Fry with Shrimp

Ingredients

- 1 head of riced cauliflower, grated or processed in a food processor a half-pound of peeled and deveined shrimp
- a variety of veggies, such as bell peppers, carrots, and peas
- 3 minced garlic cloves
- 2/fourths cup soy sauce 1/fourth cup oyster sauce one teaspoon of sesame oil chopped green onions (for garnish) pepper and salt as desired

Preparation

1. Sesame oil should be hot, and garlic should be sauteed until aromatic.

2. Cook the shrimp, stirring occasionally, until pink. Take out of the pan and place aside.

3. If more oil is required, add it to the same skillet and sauté the mixed vegetables until just tender.

4. Add cauliflower rice to the skillet after moving the vegetables to the side. Cook until well heated for a few minutes.

5. Shrimp, veggies, and cauliflower rice should all be combined. Oyster and soy sauce should be added. Stir-fry the food for a few minutes.

6. Add salt and pepper to taste.

7. Before serving, garnish with finely sliced green onions.

9.Turkey and Vegetable Skewers

Ingredients

- turkey ground or turkey breast
- various vegetables (such as cherry tomatoes, bell peppers, onions, and zucchini)
- EVOO, LEMON JUICE
- clove powder Oregano dried pepper and salt as desired

Preparation

1. Cut the turkey breast into bite-sized chunks if using. Make tiny meatballs out of ground turkey if using.

2. Make a marinade in a bowl by combining the olive oil, lemon juice, garlic powder, dried oregano, salt, and pepper.

3. Alternating between meat and vegetables, thread the turkey onto the skewers.

4. Apply the marinade on the skewers.

5. Until the turkey is thoroughly cooked and the vegetables
    are browned, grill the skewers over medium heat.

6. Along with rice or a side salad, serve the skewers hot.

10. Black Bean and Vegetable Chili

Ingredients

- 2 cans black beans, drained and rinsed one sliced onion
  2 chopped bell peppers two zucchini, cut 3 minced garlic
  cloves 1 tomato diced can one cup vegetable stock
- Chili powder, two tablespoons
- 1/9 cup cumin 1 paprika teaspoon pepper and salt as
  desired
- Almond oil
- Optional garnishes: sour cream, chopped cilantro, and
  grated cheese

Preparation

1. Olive oil should be used to sauté onions, bell peppers,
    and zucchini in a big saucepan until tender.

2. Add paprika, cumin, chili powder, and garlic. one more
    minute of cooking.

3. Add the veggie broth, diced tomatoes, and black beans.
    Simmer for a while.

4. Allow the chili to boil for 20 to 30 minutes so that the flavors can mingle and the vegetables may soften.

5. Add salt and pepper to taste.

6. Serve the chili hot with any desired additional toppings.

.

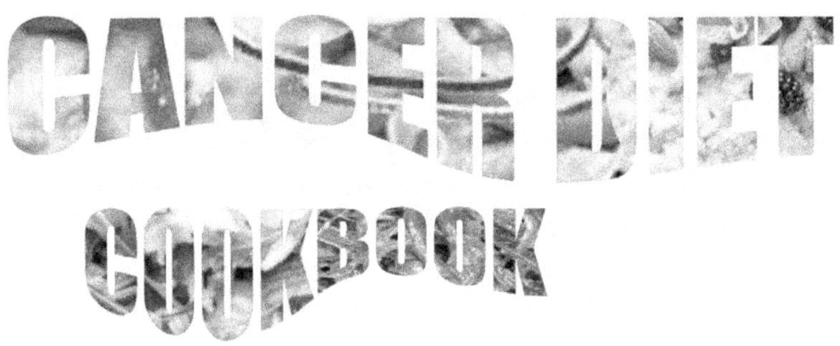

CANCER DIET
COOKBOOK *FOR* Beginners

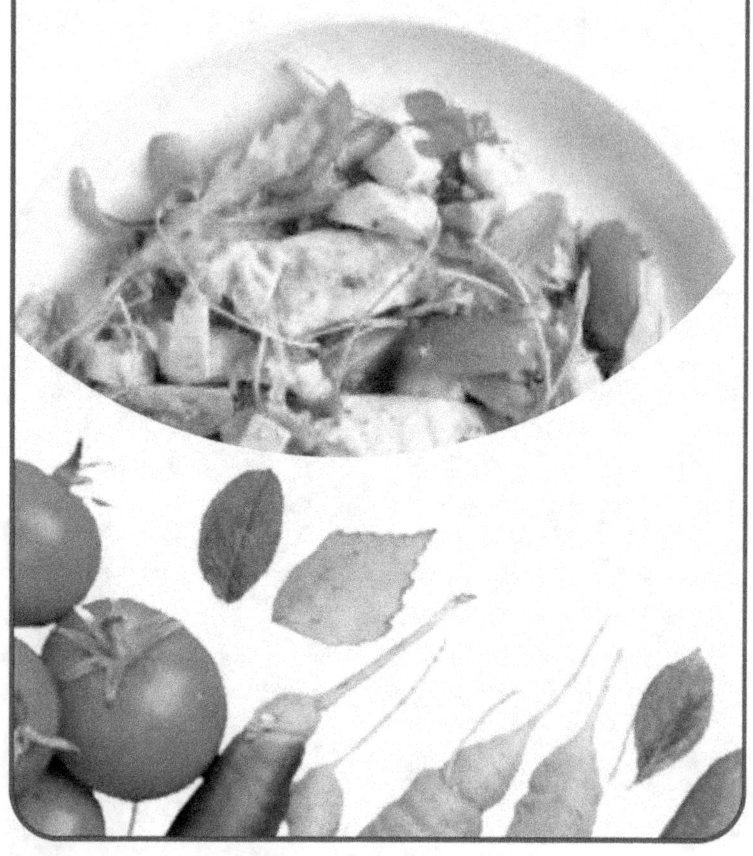

Here are 10 snack recipes suitable for a cancer-preventive or controlled diet cookbook for beginners:

1.Greek Yogurt and Berry Parfait

Ingredients

- Grecian yogurt
- Strawberries, blueberries, and raspberries mixed together (Optional) Honey or maple syrup Granola is an option.

Preparation

1. Greek yogurt should be layered at the bottom of a glass or bowl.

2. To the yogurt, add a layer of mixed berries.

3. Till the yogurt and berries are gone, keep layering.

4. If desired, drizzle with honey or maple syrup.

5. If you'd like, add some granola on top for added crunch. Enjoy the tasty and wholesome parfait!

2.Hummus and Veggie Sticks

Ingredients

- Assorted vegetables (celery, carrots, bell peppers, cucumbers, etc.) with hummus

Preparation

- The various vegetables should be washed and chopped into sticks.

- Along with a cup of hummus for dipping, offer the veggie sticks.

- Enjoy the delicious and nutritious snack by dipping the veggie sticks in the hummus!

3. Nut Butter Apple Slices

Ingredients

- Apples Nut butter, such as almond or peanut butter
- Add-ons (chia seeds, honey, and raisins)

Preparation

1. Apples should be washed and cut into rounds or wedges.

2. Each slice of apple should have a layer of nut butter on it.
3. You can choose to top the dish with chia seeds, honey, or raisins.

Enjoy the delicious fusion of creamy nut butter and crisp apples!

4. Rice Cakes with Avocado

Ingredients

- cakes of rice mature avocado pepper and salt as desired
- (Sliced tomatoes, red pepper flakes) Optional garnishes

Preparation

1. Remove the pit from the ripe avocado before scooping out the meat.

2. With a fork, mash the avocado and season with salt and
3. pepper.

4. The rice cakes should be covered with the mashed avocado. Sliced tomatoes or red pepper flakes are optional toppings.

Enjoy the light and flavorful rice cakes with avocado!

5. Trail Mix

Ingredients

- Nuts (walnuts, cashews, and other varieties)
- Dried fruits (such as apricots, raisins, and cranberries) seeds (sunflower seeds, pumpkin seeds) (Optional) Dark chocolate pieces or chips

- Popcorn or pretzels (optional)

Preparation

1. In a bowl, combine your favorite nuts, dried fruits, and seeds.

2. Add dark chocolate chunks or chips for an optional touch of sweetness.

3. You can add pretzels or popcorn for more crunch if you like.

4. After thoroughly combining all the ingredients, separate them into tiny snack bags. On the run, savor the adaptable and energizing trail mix!

6. Cottage Cheese and Pineapple

Ingredients

- Cheese cottage
- either fresh pineapple chunks or drained canned pineapple parts

Preparation

1. Into a bowl, spoon the desired amount of cottage cheese.
2. Top with fresh pineapple chunks or pineapple chunks from a can that have been drained.
3. Gently combine, then consume as a fast and protein-rich snack or small meal.

7. Kale Chips

Ingredients

- Clean and dried fresh kale leaves
- Almond oil
- Salt and seasonings (such as nutritional yeast, garlic powder, or chili powder)

Preparation:

1. Preheat the oven to 350°F (175°C).

2. The kale leaves should be stripped of their tough stems and torn into bite-sized pieces.

3. Put the chopped kale in a bowl and add little salt and olive oil to taste.

4. On a baking sheet, arrange the kale pieces in a single layer.

5. Bake the kale chips for 10 to 15 minutes, or until crisp but not burned.

6. Take them out of the oven, allow them to cool slightly, and then enjoy as a nutritious snack.

8. Oatmeal Banana Bites

Ingredients

oats in rolls mashed ripe bananas Maple syrup or honey
Cinnamon, if desired

chopped dried fruit or nuts (optional)

Preparation

1. Preheat the oven to 350°F (175°C) and line a baking sheet with parchment paper.

2. Mash some bananas, add some rolled oats, honey or maple syrup, and a little cinnamon to a bowl.

3. Add chopped nuts or dried fruit to the mixture if you'd like.

4. Shape the mixture into bite-sized rounds by scooping spoonfuls onto the baking sheet.

5. Bake the bites for 12 to 15 minutes, or until they are brown and firm.

6. Before consuming them as a pleasant and energizing

7. snack, let them cool.

9. Roasted Chickpeas

Ingredients

- Chickpeas in a can (drained and rinsed)
- Almond oil
- Paprika, cumin, garlic powder, and cayenne pepper are a few examples of seasonings.
- Salt

Preparation

1. Set the oven's temperature to 400°F (200°C).

2. With a paper towel, pat the chickpeas dry to eliminate extra moisture.

3. Put the chickpeas in a bowl and add a drizzle of olive oil, your preferred seasonings, and a bit of salt.

4. On a baking sheet, distribute the chickpeas in a single layer.

5. Roast the chickpeas until they are crispy and brown, stirring the pan every so often.

6. Before enjoying them as a crunchy, protein-rich snack, let them cool just a little.

10. Chia Seed Pudding with Berries

Ingredients

- the chia seed
- Milk (vegetable or dairy-based)
- Honey, agave syrup, or maple syrup are examples of sweeteners. Strawberries, blueberries, and raspberries: fresh berries

Preparation

- Mix the chia seeds, milk, and sweetener to taste in a bowl or jar.

- Stir thoroughly, then let the mixture rest for 10 to 15 minutes while stirring now and again. Cover the mixture and place it in the refrigerator for at least two hours or overnight once it begins to thicken.

- Give the pudding a thorough stir before serving, and then top with fresh berries.

- Take pleasure in this tasty and nourishing pudding as a delightful breakfast or dessert.

Keep in mind that you can modify these snack ideas to suit your taste preferences and dietary requirements. For individualized dietary advice, always seek the advice of a medical practitioner.

Here are 10 dessert recipes suitable for a cancer-preventive or controlled diet cookbook for beginners:

1. Mixed Berry Parfait

Ingredients

- Strawberries, blueberries, raspberries, and other mixed berries
- Grecian yogurt
- Honey or maple syrup for granola (optional)

Preparation

1. Berry cleaning and drying. Size up larger berries so that they are bite-sized.

2. Greek yogurt, mixed berries, and granola should be layered in serving glasses or bowls.

3. The layers should be repeated until the container is full.
4. If you'd like, drizzle some honey or maple syrup on top for sweetness.

2. Baked Apples with Cinnamon:

Ingredients

- apple types that are firm, such as Granny Smith and Honeycrisp the cinnamon spice
- Butter Brown sugar Chopped nuts (optional)

Preparation

Set the oven's temperature to 350°F (175°C).

1. To make a well, core the apples and take out a small portion of the center flesh.

2. In a small bowl, combine brown sugar and cinnamon.

3. Apples should be put in a baking pan. The cinnamon-sugar mixture and a small pat of butter should be added to each well.

4. Bake the apples for about 25 to 30 minutes, or until they are soft. If preferred, add chopped nuts on top just before serving.

3. Dipped Strawberries

Ingredients

*   strawberries in season
*   White, milk, dark, or a combination of these chocolates
*   (Optional) Sprinkles, chopped nuts, or coconut flakes

Preparation

1. The strawberries should be washed and completely dried.

2. Use a double boiler or a microwave to melt the chocolate while stirring to ensure smoothness.

3. Each strawberry should be dipped into the melted chocolate until roughly two-thirds of it is coated.

4. Put the strawberries on parchment paper after they have been coated.

5. If desired, quickly top with your preferred garnishes before the chocolate sets and becomes hard.

Before serving, give the chocolate time to set.

4. Chia Seed Chocolate Pudding:

Ingredients

- the chia seed
- Milk (vegetable or dairy-based) cocoa butter
- Sweetener (honey, agave, maple syrup) Vanilla flavoring

Preparation

1. Chia seeds, milk, cocoa powder, sweetener, and vanilla extract should all be combined in a bowl.

2. Make sure there are no chia seed clumps and thoroughly mix everything together. Allow the chia seeds to absorb the liquid and thicken the pudding by covering the bowl and placing it in the refrigerator for a few hours or overnight.

3. Prior to serving, stir the ingredients. If you prefer a thinner consistency, add additional milk.

5. Fruit Salad with Mint

Ingredients

- a variety of fresh fruits (oranges, grapes, kiwis, melon, pineapple, etc.) brand-new mint leaves lemon or lime juice (Optional) Honey

Preparation

1. Fruits should be washed, peeled, and diced into bite-sized pieces.

2. The diced fruits should be combined in a bowl and gently mixed.

3. Add chopped fresh mint leaves to the fruit mixture.

4. To intensify the flavors, drizzle lime or lemon juice over the fruit.

5. You might sprinkle some honey on top for added sweetness.

6. Before serving, toss everything together and place in the refrigerator for a short while.

6. Yogurt and Banana Frozen Pops

Ingredients

- two ripe bananas
- Yogurt, plain, one cup
- 2 teaspoons of maple syrup or honey Vanilla extract, 1 teaspoon

Preparation

1. Bananas, yogurt, honey (or maple syrup), and vanilla extract should all be combined in a blender.

2. Until smooth, blend.
3. Fill the popsicle molds with the mixture.

4. Popsicle sticks should be inserted and frozen for at least 4 hours, or until hard.

7. Coconut Rice Pudding

Ingredients

- Arborio rice, 1 cup coconut milk, one can
- Milk, two cups
- 1 teaspoon vanilla extract and half a cup of sugar
- A dash of salt
- Optional garnishes include cinnamon, chopped nuts, and toasted coconut flakes.

1. Arborio rice should be rinsed in cold water.

2. Combine coconut milk, milk, sugar, and salt in a pot. Simmer for a while.

3. Stir the rice after adding it to the pot.

4. Cook for 25 to 30 minutes, stirring occasionally, until the rice is tender and the stew has thickened.

5. Add vanilla extract after removing from the heat.

6. Serve warm or cold, along with any desired toppings.

8. Frozen Grapes

Ingredients

Grapes (any variety)

Preparation

1. Grapes must be washed and dried.

2. On a baking sheet, arrange the grapes in a single layer.

3. The grapes should be frozen for at least two hours, or until firm. Enjoy them as a cool and nutritious frozen snack.

9. Baked Oatmeal Cups

Ingredients

- Old-fashioned oats, 2 cups one tablespoon of baking powder half a teaspoon of cinnamon
- A dash of salt
- 1 cup milk, either dairy or vegan
- 1/4 cup honey or maple syrup
- 1 egg
- Vanilla extract, 1 teaspoon
- mixed optional-ins: chocolate chips, berries, and chopped nuts

Preparation

- Set the oven's temperature to 350°F (175°C). Either grease or line a muffin pan with paper liners.

- Oats, baking soda, cinnamon, and salt should all be combined in a bowl.

- Mix the milk, maple syrup (or honey), egg, and vanilla essence in a separate bowl.

- Mix the dry ingredients thoroughly before adding the wet ingredients.

- Add any more mix-ins by stirring.

- In the muffin cups, distribute the mixture equally.

- The tops should be brown and set after 20 to 25 minutes in the oven.

- Before removing the oatmeal cups from the tin, let them cool slightly.

10. Mango Sorbet

Ingredients

- 3 ripe mangoes, peeled and diced
- 1/4 cup sugar
- 1 tablespoon lemon or lime juice

Preparation

1. Place diced mangoes in a blender or food processor.

2. Add sugar and lemon/lime juice.

3. Blend until smooth.

4. Pour the mixture into a shallow dish and cover with plastic wrap.

5. Freeze for about 4-6 hours, or until the sorbet is firm.

6. Before serving, let the sorbet sit at room temperature for a few minutes to soften slightly. Enjoy these delicious treats!

These dessert recipes offer a healthier twist while satisfying your sweet cravings. Adjust them according to your preferences and dietary requirements.

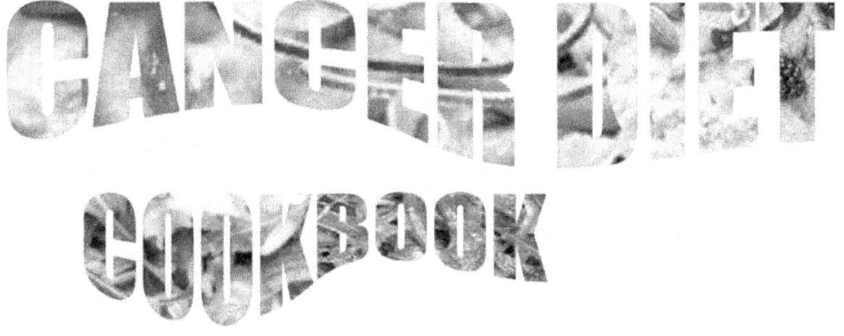

Sure, here's a 28-day meal plan using the breakfast, lunch, dinner, snacks, and dessert recipes you provided:

Week 1:

Day 1
Breakfast: Oatmeal with Berries
Lunch: Grilled Chicken Salad
Dinner: Baked Salmon with Steamed Vegetables
Snack: Greek Yogurt and Berry Parfait
Dessert: Mixed Berry Parfait

Day 2
Breakfast: Greek Yogurt Parfait
Lunch: Quinoa and Vegetable Stir-Fry
Dinner: Grilled Chicken with Quinoa and Roasted Veggies
Snack: Hummus and Veggie Sticks
Dessert: Baked Apples with Cinnamon

Day 3
Breakfast: Avocado Toast
Lunch: Mediterranean Wrap
Dinner: Stir-Fried Tofu and Broccoli
Snack: Nut Butter Apple Slices
Dessert: Chocolate-Dipped Strawberries

Breakfast: Spinach and Mushroom Scramble
Lunch: Tomato Basil Soup
Dinner: Whole-Wheat Pasta with Tomato and Basil Sauce
Snack: Rice Cakes with Avocado
Dessert: Chia Seed Chocolate Pudding

Day 5

Breakfast: Quinoa Breakfast Bowl
Lunch: Lentil Salad
Dinner: Baked Sweet Potato with Black Beans and Salsa
Snack: Trail Mix
Dessert: Fruit Salad with Mint

Day 6

Breakfast: Chia Seed Pudding
Lunch: Brown Rice Bowl with Salmon
Dinner: Veggie and Lentil Stew
Snack: Cottage Cheese and Pineapple
Dessert: Yogurt and Banana Frozen Pops

Day 7

Breakfast: Smoked Salmon Wrap
Lunch: Chickpea and Vegetable Curry
Dinner: Grilled Veggie and Hummus Wrap
Snack: Kale Chips
Dessert: Coconut Rice Pudding

Week 2-4: Follow the same pattern as Week 1, rotating through the various breakfast, lunch, dinner, snack, and dessert options provided.

Remember that this is just a sample meal plan and you can mix and match the recipes based on your preferences and nutritional needs. It's important to ensure a balanced intake of nutrients and calories to maintain a healthy diet.

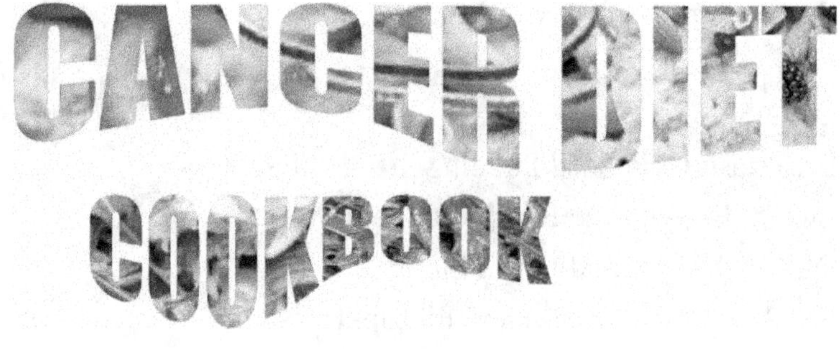

CONCLUSION

In conclusion, this cookbook serves as a guiding light for those embarking on a journey towards a cancer-preventive or controlled diet. It has been meticulously crafted to empower beginners with a wealth of diverse and delectable recipes, each thoughtfully designed to align with the principles of a health-conscious lifestyle.

Throughout these pages, you've discovered a harmonious fusion of flavors, textures, and ingredients that not only tantalize the taste buds but also nourish the body in ways that promote well-being. From the breakfast table to dinnertime, and every snack and dessert in between, this cookbook has aimed to cater to your cravings while maintaining a steadfast commitment to your health.

In your hands lies a treasure trove of culinary creations that prioritize the power of wholesome ingredients, mindful preparation, and balanced nutrition. By embracing the recipes contained within these pages, you're embracing a lifestyle that has the potential to be a shield against cancer and other health challenges.

Remember, this cookbook is not just a collection of recipes; it's a roadmap to a more vibrant and resilient you. The journey to a healthier you begins here, and it is our hope that these recipes become your trusted companions along the way. As you savor each bite, may you find inspiration, fulfillment, and a renewed sense of purpose in the pursuit of a healthier, cancer-preventive path.

Here's to your well-being, your culinary adventures, and a future defined by vitality and joy. Let these recipes be a testament to the incredible potential that lies within the choices we make for our plates and, ultimately, our lives. Your journey has just begun, and with this cookbook as your guide, the path to a healthier future is rich with delicious possibilities

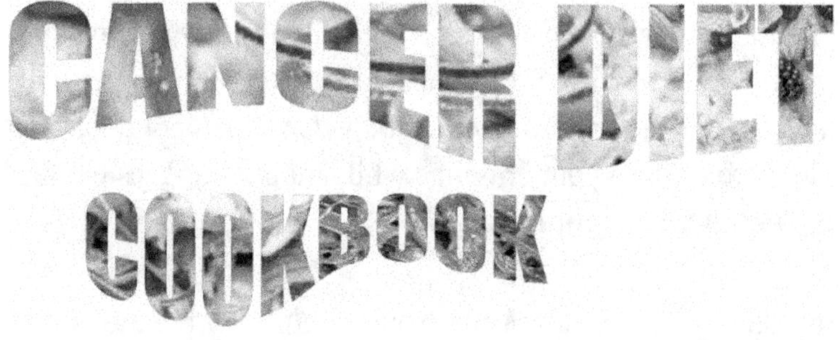

Thank you for embarking on this culinary voyage with us, exploring the pages of this cookbook dedicated to a cancer-preventive or controlled diet. Your commitment to learning, embracing, and implementing these health-conscious recipes is a testament to your dedication to well-being.

As you close the final chapter of this book, we extend our heartfelt gratitude for your time and trust. Your willingness to explore new flavors, experiment in the kitchen, and prioritize your health is truly commendable. By delving into these recipes, you've not only enriched your own journey but also demonstrated a profound commitment to making informed, positive choices for your body and future.

May your culinary adventures continue to blossom, and may the knowledge and inspiration you've gained here serve as a foundation for a vibrant and resilient life. Remember, every ingredient you choose and every dish you create holds the potential to shape your well-being in powerful ways.

Thank you for your curiosity, your determination, and your unwavering dedication to a healthier and more fulfilling lifestyle. May your path be sprinkled with health, happiness, and the joy of nourishing your body and spirit. Here's to you, your health, and the countless delicious possibilities that lie ahead

14 DAY MEAL PLANNER

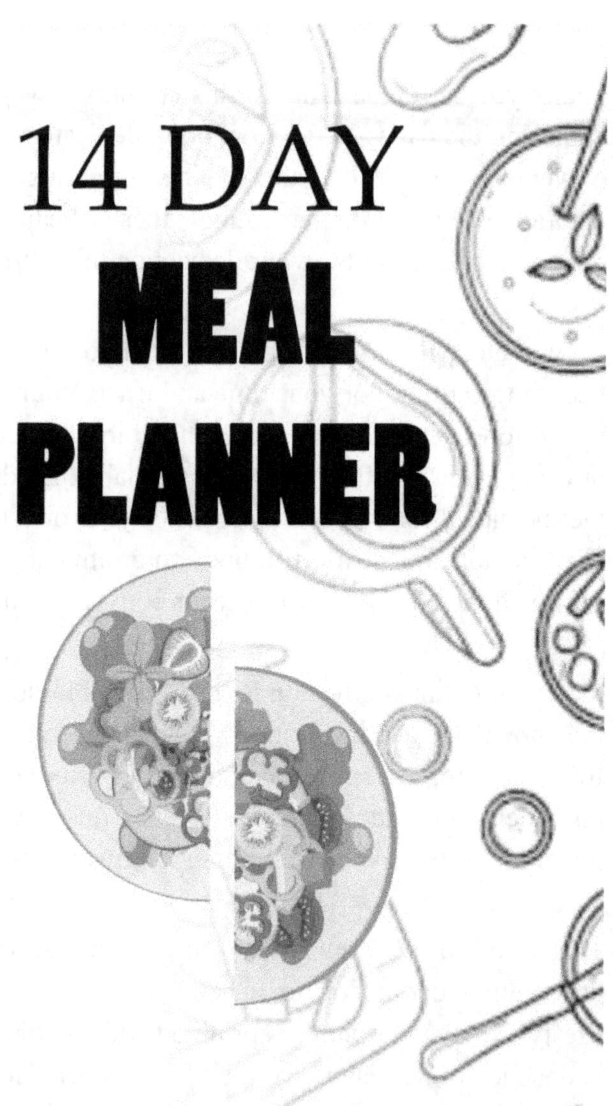

Menu List:

Breakfast

Lunch

Dinner

Important Meal:

shopping list:

To Do List

Notes And Tips

Breakfast

Lunch

Dinner

Important Meal;

shopping list:

To Do List

Notes And Tips

Menu List:

Breakfast

Lunch

Dinner

Important Meal:

shopping list:

To Do List

....

....

....

....

....

● ....

● ....

● ....

● ....

● ....

Notes And Tips   TO DO

Breakfast

Lunch

Dinner

Important Meal:

shopping list:

To Do List

Notes And Tips

Menu List:

Breakfast

Lunch

Dinner

Important Meal:

shopping list:

To Do List

Notes And Tips   TO DO

Menu List:

Breakfast

Lunch

Dinner

Important Meal:

shopping list:

To Do List

Notes And Tips

Menu List:

Breakfast

Lunch

Dinner

Important Meal:

shopping list:

To Do List

Notes And Tips

Menu List:

Breakfast

Lunch

Dinner

Important Meal:

shopping list:

To Do List

....
....
....
....
....

Notes And Tips

Menu List:

Breakfast

Lunch

Dinner

Important Meal:

shopping list:

To Do List

Notes And Tips

Menu List:

Breakfast

Lunch

Dinner

Important Meal:

shopping list:

To Do List

Notes And Tips

Menu List:

Breakfast

Lunch

Dinner

Important Meal;

shopping list:

To Do List

Notes And Tips

Menu List:

Breakfast

Lunch

Dinner

Important Meal:

shopping list:

To Do List

Notes And Tips

Menu List:

Breakfast

Lunch

Dinner

Important Meal:

shopping list:

To Do List

Notes And Tips

Menu List:

Breakfast

Lunch

Dinner

Important Meal:

shopping list:

To Do List

Notes And Tips

Menu List:

Breakfast

Lunch

Dinner

Important Meal:

shopping list:

To Do List

Notes And Tips

Menu List:

Breakfast

Lunch

Dinner

Important Meal;

shopping list:

To Do List

Notes And Tips

Menu List:

Breakfast

Lunch

Dinner

Important Meal:

shopping list:

To Do List

Notes And Tips

Menu List:

Breakfast

Lunch

Dinner

Important Meal;

To Do List

shopping list:

Notes And Tips